COGNITIVE BEHAVIORAL THERAPY

INTRODUCTION

CBT tends to deal with the 'here and now'-how you are now affecting your current thoughts and behaviours. It recognizes that events in your past have shaped the way you currently think and behave, particularly in childhood learning thought patterns and behaviors. CBT does not, however, dwell on the past, but aims at finding solutions to change your current thoughts and behaviors so you can function better in the future.

The therapy is based on the simple idea that the way we think directly affects our behaviour, so also our behavior and reaction to situations or events will be irrational when we have irrational or distorted thoughts and perceptions. During CBT sessions, the psychiatrist splits up issues into small pieces, which can be addressed one at a time very quickly. The starting point is a specific situation or event; then the immediate, flawed thoughts of the person on that situation are examined. These mistaken thoughts, often negative, lead the person to have certain emotions and physical feelings, which in turn prompts them to react and act in a negative, unhelpful manner. A trained CBT therapist aims to change the thinking patterns of the patient by demonstrating how much more helpful, rational and positive are their emotions and resulting behaviors when their initial thoughts are correct, realistic and rational.

Clinical trials suggest that CBT has been successful in tackling different emotional issues. Research studies have shown, for example, that a course of CBT is just as effective in treating depression and some anxiety disorders as medication. It is also possible that the effects of CBT will continue to protect the client against further illness in the longer term. People who finish medication may be at higher risk of relapse compared with CBT clients who have learned principles and strategies to sustain their recovery, so problems such as depression or anxiety are less likely to recur in the future, for example. There is also good evidence of research showing that CBT can help improve the symptoms of some physical conditions such as rheumatoid arthritis.

CHAPTER ONE

CBT for Anxiety Disorder

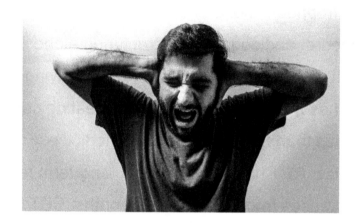

BT, especially in vivo exposure, obtains the most reliable outcomes for the treatment of severe phobias, but it is correlated with high dropout levels and poor approval of therapy. So it may be desirable to combine the cognitive and behavioral components. Cognitive restructuring is effective in the treatment of claustrophobia alone and in combination with in vivo exposure, and cognitive restructuring alone is effective in the treatment of dental and flying phobias. CBT has more positive effects for treating common phobias than hypnotherapy and medicine. For certain phobias, CBT has demonstrated long-term retention of increases from 12.0 to 13.8 months. CBT demonstrates mild to strong total efficacy for overcoming social phobia. The most common combination of CBT components is cognitive rehabilitation plus stimulation, but inconsistent results make the dominance of this combination over other combinations, or solo elements, uncertain. One analysis showed CBT by itself and CBT plus pharmacotherapy were similarly successful. Complicating the data is the fact that each study defines CBT and exposure differently. However, community CBT is the most cost-effective and tolerable therapy, and the medication of choice for social phobia should also be considered. CBT's long-term success for social phobia has been proven for up to 12 months.

The total efficacy of CBT is overwhelming and well-supported for OCD. Cognitive therapy and ERP are two aspects of well-defined CBT strategies which are frequently merged. No support is given for the incremental benefit of adding cognitive techniques to BT; typically, BT outperforms CBT. However, cognitive approaches improve therapy tolerability, inspire clients and help them control the elements dependent on sensitivity. Aside from BT, CBT has not been compared to other psychotherapies. There has not been a clear contrast of pharmacotherapy and CBT and definitive conclusions can not be made. A limited volume of evidence suggests that any medication alone may be preferable to a mixture of pharmacotherapy and CBT. Insufficient data are available to report on the continued efficacy of CBT, and to distinguish between PD and PDA performance.

CBT 's controlled and unchecked absolute efficacy for PD / PDA has been amply demonstrated. Exposure and cognitive restructuring are the typical constituents of CBT for PD / PDA. Adding cognitive components to behavioral components for PD / PDA treatment does not result in incremental value in terms of reduced anxiety, but in terms of reduced symptoms of depression and attrition rates. CT is superior to RT but no other comparisons have been reviewed between psychotherapies and CBT. There is a mix of evidence for the relative effectiveness of pharmacotherapy and CBT; some studies have considered the two to be similarly effective; some have reported divergent outcomes based on the outcome factors examined; and others have found proof of CBT dominance over pharmacotherapy. There are also mixed results with respect to the relative efficacy of CBT alone and a combined intervention in CBT – pharmacotherapy. Lastly, CBT has the best cost profile of the interventions, and the long-term effectiveness of CBT has been demonstrated up to 16.8 months on average. Chronic PTSD has received the most research attention, but the literature on CBT treatment efficacy has also examined immediate post-trauma experiences and acute PTSD. TFCBT (that is, exposure and trauma-focused cognitive techniques) is the most widely studied form of CBT. TFCBT and EMDR both have demonstrated controlled absolute efficacy for chronic PTSD, are superior to "other therapies," and are not significantly different from one another. TFCBT can only be considered tentatively superior to pharmacotherapy (i.e., paroxetine) for the treatment of chronic PTSD, due to limited and inconclusive evidence. CBT 's controlled absolute efficacy for GAD treatment is well-established for the short term; however, due to insufficient data, long-term results are indeterminate. Compared with CBT, the relative efficacy of pharmacotherapy is not clear; the data is inconsistent, based on the particular effects measured. For at least one study, however, scholars surmised that CBT is better tolerated than pharmacotherapy. CBT has shown dominance over post-treatment and 6-month follow-up psychodynamic intervention, modest dominance over positive intervention, inconsistent outcomes relative to BT, and comparable effectiveness compared to RT. In the meta-analyses we reviewed, the relative effectiveness of CBT compared to combined CBT and pharmacotherapy was not stated. CBT for GAD recovery literature covers several aspects under the CBT rubric, including instruction in anxiety reduction, cognitive rehabilitation, acute awareness, self-controlled desensitization, RT/reading, CT alone, and BT alone.

At this point, cognitive behavioral therapy (CBT) could be the leading choice for treating many forms of anxiety. This has been found to be as effective in treating panic disorder and phobias as prescription drugs, and it also shows considerable potential for treating obsessive-compulsive disorder and post-traumatic stress disorder. It's not a "wonder drug," or magic cure, however. Cognitive behavioural therapy for the diagnosis of anxiety illness is a relatively complicated procedure that often involves ongoing and patient constructive involvement, as well as instruction in most cases by a professional teacher or therapist.

For starters, cognitive behavioral therapy is not one thing, but rather a general term for a number of similar but distinct therapies, such as Rational Emotional Behavior Therapy, Rational Behavior Therapy, Rational Living Therapy, Cognitive Therapy, and Dialectic Behavior Therapy.

However, one thing all these therapies share is the belief that what actually controls our feelings and behaviors is our thoughts — not external things like people, situations, and events. And if we can change the way we think, even if the external factors do not change, we can feel better and react differently. The role of the therapist is to teach the clients how to recognize and challenge and consciously correct their own irrational and self-destructive beliefs.

CBT is an educational process that holds that they can be unlearned to the extent that emotional and behavioral reactions are learned. The purpose of counseling is to help clients unlearn unhealthy responses and replace them with new ways of responding to sources of stress and anxiety.

CBT therapists are focused on teaching rational self-control skills. Counseling sessions rely on conversation and structured interviews to help patients identify the specific thoughts and situations that disturb them, rationally analyze those factors, and learn specific techniques and concepts to defuse them when they grow. Homework and reading tasks are an integral part of the process and are crucial to making CBT a therapy that is fairly short-term and time-limited.

Homework and techniques commonly used in CBT include keeping a diary of events and the feelings, thoughts and behaviors that they trigger; asking questions and challenging the faulty or unrealistic perceptions and beliefs of the patient; learning to overcome avoidance and confront challenging situations and activities; training in techniques of relaxation, mindfulness and distraction.

Exposure therapy and desensitization for anxiety disorders are essential features of most CBTs. Once the client and therapist have identified the triggers of anxiety and their associated feelings and thoughts, they work to break the pattern of response by recreating or evoking those events and feelings under controlled conditions. Starting by teaching calming methods, meditation, or breathing exercises that will help the patient to manage their apprehension and anxiety during the exposure phase is important. Gradual repetitive conditions cause the patient to cope with reduced stress thresholds and gradually build up until he or she is no longer responsive to the previous stimuli.

CBT is a technique that is deeply empowering and is one reason why it is so effective in treating anxiety-related disorders. Understanding the relationship between your mental and physical symptoms and knowing that you have tools and techniques to manage these symptoms can significantly reduce anticipatory anxiety-which is often the key difference between occasional disturbing but essentially normal episodes of anxiety or even panic, and a full-blown chronic anxiety disorder that weakens.

How Can CBT Eliminate Your anxiety Attacks?

Many of us agree that the circumstances we encounter and our everyday encounters are the causes of fear, panic, and depression. For example, if you drive your car, and you get an anxiety attack when you get on a highway, you probably think your anxiety is caused by driving up the highway. In not true, this. According to CBT the intensity of your emotions is determined by your thoughts and set of beliefs.

Cognitive behavioural therapy gives you easy strategies to avoid dead episodes of fear and anxiety in their path.

CBT is the only method that can permanently cure anxiety and panic disorder, because it uses scientifically verified strategies to relieve long-term anxiety. Other popular treatments — such as medication, herbal remedies, breathing exercises, and more — usually only treat symptoms of anxiety and don't treat the root of the problem — your brain and your thinking!

Cognitive Behavioral Therapy for Treatment of Anxiety Disorder

Cognitive-behavioral therapy, or CBT, works on the minds and behaviors of the patient to change how they feel and how they react to "negative" situations. CBT is based on the assumption that the way we react to things is conditioned, and that the conditioned responses can be changed by unlearning them.

CBT aims to identify the patterns of thinking that negatively affect the life of the patient, and to find more resourceful ways of thinking or self-talking. Examples of distorted mindsets include:

• Should / must think: turn your interests and desires into pure necessities. Some examples of this kind of thinking include: "I have to get this," "this shouldn't have happened," "this person should have been nice to me."

• Overgeneralization: you see a single unwanted event as a permanent pattern of malaise. For instance: somebody doesn't treat you well and you think "I can never please people," even though the other person has treated you badly because he or she wasn't in good mood.

• Magnification and minimisation: the negatives are exaggerated and the positive discounted. You 're driving and turning in the wrong direction for starters. Then you think: "I have a terrible sense of direction" or "I'm such a bad driver," even if you rarely make this kind of "mistake."

• Mind-reading: You assume what others think of you without having any real evidence of your assumption.

We can see that such thought forms cause anxiety. Within you, you may find these patterns of thought to be factual , accurate or essential. Yet you don't have to look at them like this. We also see other people around us who act appropriately and do well in the circumstances outlined in the scenarios mentioned above, even when these situations happen far more times to these individuals than we would find reasonable individually. The way we respond is more about our programmed responses and values than anything else.

CBT therapy is reciprocal, as the patient has to apply the strategies suggested by the psychiatrist in their everyday lives. The patient's activities may include writing down a list of the feelings , emotions and habits that happened in the patient's everyday life following traumatic events. The therapist will evaluate this list to determine distorted thoughts and more resourceful ways to tackle the particular issue. The therapy may also involve (gradual) imaginary exposure to a situation of fear or phobia, or exposure to real life.

The cause of the problem is not relevant for CBT, because it focuses on the "here and how," i.e., the thoughts and behaviors that cause the problem or contribute to it.

Although, other types of psychotherapy may take years for the benefits to come, CBT treatment usually lasts a couple of months.

Cure Your Anxiety Condition with CBT

The wide range of anxiety conditions, including panic disorder, obsessive compulsive disorder, post-traumatic stress disorder, generalized anxiety disorder, social anxiety disorder, and phobias, are permanently cured. Anxiety disorders plague 40 million American adults, ages 18 and older, according to the National Institute for Mental Health (NIMH). As we mull over the meaning of this staggering number, let 's look at the recommended treatment method, one that provides recovery for hundreds of thousands of patients.

Cognitive behavioural therapy is in essence a fusion of two separate approaches, all of which trace their origins back to the 1950s and 1960s — and their adoption by the psychiatric community during the 1970s and 1980s.

The American psychiatrist Aaron T. Beck developed cognitive therapy during the 1960's. Beck initially applied his approach to depression issues, then broadened his practice to include anxiety disorders. How it is that people interpret and assign meaning to their everyday lives is a process called cognition. Beck, disillusioned with conventional psychotherapeutic delving into the subconscious, believed that perception was the secret to successful treatment and would lead to meaningful healing, as his patients understood it.

Beck first found, while designing his treatment, that suicidal individuals embrace a pessimistic view of the environment during formative years — based on the death of a loved one, social disappointment, criticism by sources of power, depressive behaviors present in other important ones, plus a host of spontaneous adverse incidents. Very commonly, a distorted, subjective view of the world reinforces and nurtures this negative perception — for example, all-or-nothing thought, overgeneralization, and narrow beliefs that ignore important, concrete facts. Cognitive therapy postulates that distortions grow to disorders in a person's perspectives. It is a cognitive therapist's job to point these distortions out and to encourage change in the attitude of a sufferer.

Beginning in 1953, in the United States, behaviour modification made its debut in a groundbreaking effort led by B.F. Skinner. Skinner. In South Africa, the credit for pioneering work goes to Joseph Wolpe and his research group. Hans Eysenck has contributed to the development of such therapy in the United Kingdom.

Behavioral therapy is mainly based on functional analysis. Behavioral therapies have been used widely as a treatment for disorders of marriage, physical pain, fatigue, anorexia, psychological illness, drug misuse, psychiatric depression and anxiety.

Behavioral therapy focuses on the environment and its context and is data-driven and contextual. Behavioral therapy generally concerns the effect or outcome of behavior, behavior is regarded as objectively predictable; a person is handled as an individual without the complications of a mind-to-body approach, but partnerships, bidirectional experiences, are well taken into consideration.

The anxiety conditions were originally considered to be by-products of chemical imbalances and/or genetic predispositions. With those notions abandoned, learned behaviors were credited as the source of most conditions of anxiety. There was hope for a permanent cure, and cognitive therapy and behavioral therapy merged into cognitive behavioral therapy (CBT) in the 1990s. The common ground for these two therapies is to emphasize the "here and now" by focusing on symptom alleviation and replacing harmful, self-destructive behavior with beneficial beliefs and attitudes.

In the UK , the National Centre for Health and Professional Excellence proposes CBT as the best therapy for mental health issues such as OCD, post-traumatic stress disorder, bulimia, severe depression, and even chronic fatigue syndrome for the neurological condition. In the United States, CBT has gained recognition within the medical community, given our fascination with prescription solutions. Skilled, outcome-driven help is available to those who are seeking it.

CHAPTER TWO

CBT and Psychotherapy Integration

One of conflict and change, is the history of psychotherapy. The evolution of theory and practice has been both the product and the precipitator of rivalry and disagreement between those who instigate change and those who support the day's accepted theory. Early theories evolved largely through disagreements among the "talking cure" practitioners. Freud's disciples broke with him due to disagreements concerning both the nature of psychopathology and treatment techniques. Such disjunctive progress, in any new field, is understandable. Since research studies are scarce and the main means of exploration (as in early psychotherapy) are by unregulated experiments (e.g., patient case analysis), improvements in the field are eventually influenced by political discord and perception discrepancies.

Particularly in the early history of psychotherapy, the disputes that existed between theorists and practitioners were based inextricably on the fundamental issue of what constitutes proof of reality. Theoretical positions on psychotherapy have become sacrosanct, and scientific findings have been rejected because they have not fit the canons of one theoretical position or another. That situation created Babel 's virtual tower, and theories developed during the 1970s with unchecked abandonment. When the proliferation of different theoretical viewpoints reached its zenith in the 1980s, it would have been difficult to find any position on the nature or effectiveness of psychotherapy that would gain consensus, let alone the majority.

While the remnants of this discord remain, scientific findings are more acceptable than previously, and "evidence-based practice" has become the norm in medicine and other health care professions. Scientific inquiry and evidence derived through the scientific method gained ground as agents of change for the field. The disputes that emerge among practitioners, and between academic and practitioner cultures, discuss the importance of empirical evidence as knowledge baseless frequently than what constitutes "good" research. Most psychotherapists accept the value of scientific enquiry, at least in principle, even though they differ widely in what they consider acceptable scientific methods. However, despite this development, the acceptance of scientific findings as the basis for setting new directions or for deciding what is factual among practitioner therapists has been decidedly lagging. Indeed for many practitioners, the true test of a given psychotherapy rests on the observations of clinicians in both its theoretical logic and evidence, rather than data from sound scientific methods, even when the latter are available.

What practitioners accept as valid depends on both the methods and the strength of their opinions used to derive results. Practitioners prefer naturalistic research to randomized clinical studies, N = 1 or single-case studies to group designs, and individualization to group outcome measures. They also prefer to accept research that promotes the model they use over research that advocates alternate approaches to psychotherapy, or equivalence between methods. Since most research into psychotherapy fails to meet these values, psychotherapists are often quick to reject scientific findings that disagree with their own theoretical systems. So while the reasons given for rejecting scientific evidence may today be more sophisticated than in the past, it may not be less likely to happen.

The Emergence of Eclectic and Integrationist Views

Theorists who distance themselves from a mentor 's beliefs have also been viewed as pariahs. Consequently, it was not unusual to find that a practitioner of a particular theoretical orientation was quite ignorant of other theoretical schools' principles and practices. While this theoretical isolation may have motivated therapists and clinicians to refine and enhance the skills and techniques embraced by their respective theoretical orientations, its horizons and perspectives are also severely limited.

The psychotherapy field has evolved since the 1980s, in reaction to the rise of integrationist and multicultural views. This change was partially stimulated by the diversity of field opinion and the status of scientific evidence.

With over 400 different theories about the landscape of psychotherapy, the inescapable conclusion was that there was no single truth about psychopathology or psychotherapy. Practitioners were wary of theory and a profound disaffection for specific theoretical orientations grew. Dissatisfaction was compounded by the failure of scientific studies to firmly indicate any psychotherapy 's clear superiority relative to the others. Indeed, research showed that none of the psychotherapies adequately produced the systematic approaches that would contribute to the effective treatment of patients dealing with difficult and severe problems. Over the last few years, physicians have adopted ideas, strategies, and approaches from different fields of thought in an attempt to improve their own overall therapeutic efficacy.

Although the eclectic and integrationist movement caught on in the 1980s, its nucleus was in Thorne (1962), and Goldstein and Stein (1976) early works. Thorne's "eclectic" psychotherapy arose in counseling theory from a relational perspective. He argued that training doomed therapists to a single-method perspective that was inadequate to the variety of conditions, personalities, and needs of different patients, in much the same way that a carpenter who only had a screwdriver would be inadequately equipped to build a home. Thorne gave a diverse philosophical case with little basic institutional instructions. Goldstein and Stein, on the other hand, suggested that the selected procedures should be based on scientific evidence of effectiveness, and they presented examples of evidence-based treatments. Because of their scientific bent, these latter recommendations were largely derived from the literature on behavioral therapy, since at that point in time, behaviorism was the dominant approach in research. Modern eclecticism has become wider in scope but retained some of the values inherent in Thorne 's acceptance of procedures from a variety of perspectives, and in Goldstein and Stein's admonition to let scientific evidence dictate the methods of application rather than theory.

Surveys indicate that most North American mental health professionals identify with some form of eclecticism, or what is more commonly referred to as "integration," since the term implies a systematic application of concepts and techniques spawned by a variety of psychotherapies and pathology theories. As documented by membership of the Society for the Exploration of Psychotherapy Integration (SEPI), growth in the integrationist movement is international in scale.

Within the integrationist movement, at least four perspectives can be identified (Goldfried, 1995; Norcross & Goldfried, 1992; Norcross, Martin, Omer, & Pinsoff, 1996):

(1) Common Eclectic Factors,

(2) Theoretical inclusionism,

(3) and technological eclecticism;

(4) The eclecticism of a strategy.

Besides the unsystematic form of "haphazard eclecticism" to which many practitioners adhere, these approaches do exist. Haphazard eclecticism is based on some of the common convictions and statistical "evidence" that define the diverse tradition's more formal trends, most prominently the objective finding that different methods tend to be better tailored to different individuals. Unsystematic eclecticism, however, does not define the principles governing the merging of points of view, or a replicable procedure for selecting and applying treatments. This approach to eclecticism is widespread, but its effectiveness is hard to assess, as it varies between therapists as well as within them. Its effectiveness is inextricably bound up with the judgment and abilities of the therapist in question who applies it.

"Common factors eclecticism" relies among the more formal approaches on factors which are popular or close across approaches. The common psychotherapy approach to factors is different from the way one usually thinks about eclecticism. Common eclecticism factors accept that all effective psychotherapies are based on a core of basic ingredients, beyond which their distinctive effects are inconsistent or unpredictable. This approach seeks to recognize strategies or behaviors that occur in all effective therapies, and suggests that studies should examine the approaches and psycho-therapeutic relationships that facilitate or involve certain specific causes or attributes. This posture suggests that these common interventions will comprise effective psychotherapy.

The therapist working within the growing approach to causes is never associated with particular approaches or methods, except those resulting in a congenial and loving partnership. Common therapist factors, such as most relationship-oriented therapists, create an accepting and non-threatening atmosphere in which the patient can explore problems. But unlike relationship-oriented therapies driven by specific psychopathology theories and changes, a certain type of therapy relationship is considered necessary and sufficient, and no more specific techniques or procedures are considered useful.

Though common factors are important elements of change, the contribution of specific classes of treatment interventions is supported by a growing research body. For example, recent research with manualized alcoholism treatments for cognitive — behavioral and family systems delivered in a couple format has suggested that both common treatment elements and specific interventions contribute to change. More specifically, components of the treatment appear to operate in a complex manner, independently and/or in interaction. In addition, the balance of common to specific elements of treatment exerts positive or attenuating effects depending on the treatment phase, the type of treatment given and the time of follow-up after treatment.

The preponderance of systematic eclectic hypotheses tackles the nature and variation of patients and therapies (aptitude x clinical experiences, or ATIs) by structuring and systematizing prescribed therapeutic interventions, since optimizing access to this particular mix of therapeutic variables better reduces the difficulties of patients (Stricker & Gold, 1996). These initiatives are driven at one end by what is termed "abstract integrationism" and at the other end by "scientific eclecticism." Among these poles are the conceptual eclectics, which combine all abstract ideas and methods at the level of behavioral effect action approaches and values. All three approaches are more systematic than either haphazard eclecticism, or common eclecticism factors. They share a common goal of guiding the therapist through decisions on which procedures to apply, who, and when. They identify the range of procedures to be used, and the patient or temporal and situational indications that index their maximum impact point. The theoretical integration movement, at the broadest level, attempts to amalgamate at least two theoretical viewpoints but leaves the specific techniques and procedures to the judgment of the clinician. These approaches see good theory as the avenue for developing good techniques; they contrast those approaches, which are often referred to in nature as either "eclectic" or "strategic."

The term "integration" has a set of meanings that go beyond the psychotherapy theories of interdigitation. For example, when you refer to an integrated personality in which the component traits, needs, wants, perceptions, values, emotions, and impulses are in a stable state of harmony and communication, it can refer to the quality of one's personality. An integrated person is one who is entire in terms of overall functioning and well-being. Integration in psychotherapy requires harmonious attempts to link affective, emotional, therapeutic, and program approaches to psychotherapy under a common framework, and to apply this philosophy to the treatment of people, groups, and families. This notion goes beyond any single theory or set of techniques and incorporates various models of human working. Theoretical integration requires, at least superficially, the translation of concepts and methods from one psycho-therapeutic system into the language and procedures of another. What always comes up is a new idea that incorporates elements of each of the previous ones. This theory encompasses identifying and standardizing effective concepts, terms and methods, and includes applying the resulting theoretical concepts to the research and application grist mill. Theoretical linkages among psychodynamic, behavioral, and cognitive approaches were made using an integration system. Theoretical integration is the most abstract theoretical of the various systemic approaches. Theoretical integration attempts to bring together different theories through the development of a theoretical framework that can explain an individual's environmental, motivational, cognitive and affective domains that influence or are influenced by efforts to change; that is, theoretical integrative approaches combine two or more traditional theoretical orientations to produce a new person model Ideally these new forms of therapy capitalize on the strengths of each of the therapeutic elements. Technical and strategic eclecticism is often seen as more clinically oriented and practical than theoretical integration. Strategic and technical approaches to eclectic therapy are less abstract than theoretical models of integration, and rely more on the utilization of specific techniques , procedures or principles. They define a variety of strategies (strategic eclecticism) or develop menus of psychotherapeutic interventions (technical eclecticism), irrespective of the theory which gave rise to these procedures. These types of integration are accomplished through a neutral perspective on the theories of change, or the adoption of a super-ordinate theory to replace or supersede the originals.

Technical and political eclectics are mainly concerned with the therapeutic efficacy of therapy methods, and do not pay any attention to the nature of the psychopathology and temperament hypotheses that give rise to these methods. These eclectics employ interventions from two or more psychotherapeutic systems and apply them to patients who have indicated qualities systematically and successively, using guidelines or heuristics based either on demonstrated or presumed clinical efficacy. This does not mean that the approaches in the technical eclectic tradition are devoid of theory; however, to the extent that theories are used, they are theories that link numerous empirical observations and rarely require the level of abstractness inherent in most traditional therapeutic change theories.

Multimodal therapy is the first and best known of the technically eclectic approaches (MMT; Lazarus, 1996). Around the same time, or in a structured series, MMT therapists apply various psychological methods and models based on the relative significance of the patient's symptoms. In other forms of technical eclecticism, prescriptive matching is dedicated to integrating a host of specific procedures, chosen from a wide range of menus, into a coherent and seamless treatment.

In the specificity of recommended procedures and techniques, the major distinction between technical eclecticism and strategic eclecticism is. Technical eclecticism provides a set of procedures that would suit a single individual or issue. Strategic eclecticism, by contrast, defines values and objectives but leaves the collection of approaches to the particular therapist's proclivities. The tacit or operating principle of technological eclecticism is that all techniques have a limited spectrum of applicability and application, whereas strategic eclecticism believes that all techniques can be employed in different forms and for different purposes, based on whether and by whom they are used.

Strategic therapy offers a middle ground between the technical emphasis of technological eclecticism and the theoretical integrationism abstract. Those approaches articulate therapeutic change principles that lead to general intervention strategies. The strategies are designed to implement the guiding principles, but the aim is to remain true to the principles rather than just focus on the specific techniques. As such, these approaches preserve individual therapist's flexibility in selecting particular techniques. They also maximize the use of techniques that are familiar and skilled to the therapist, without forgetting to use patient factors as reliable indicators for the selective application of various interventions. Typically such approaches provide clear interpretation of guiding principles that promote values of relationships, and elicit symptomatic and systemic changes. And they are perhaps the most versatile and realistic of the various approaches to integration: not as nuanced and comprehensive as integrationist approaches, and not as simple as technological eclecticism.

Though prescriptive psychotherapy sometimes resembles technical eclecticism, by constructing principles of change, it goes beyond the latter. The aim is a coherent treatment based on an overall view of the patient's presentation. Treatments based on explicit principles of change, such as those based on elaborate psychopathology theories, are most usefully integrated if researchable, do not rely on abstract concepts for which there is no measurement, and place few theory-driven bans on the use of various therapeutic techniques.

While most systematic eclectic psychotherapies span multiple theories, others use principles to guide the utilization of specific theories. Cognitive therapy (CT), for example, is appropriate for the application of diverse concepts since it focuses on scientific results rather than theoretical causal hypotheses and emphasizes accurate assessment of individual characteristics, improvement and recovery methods. For efficacy in the therapeutic arena, CT does not depend on the validity of insights into the nature of psychopathology In the assessment of treatment effects, cognitive theory first and foremost emphasizes reliable observation and measurement.

Thus, cognitive theory offers a platform from which one could begin to integrate change principles and strategic definition that includes, but is not limited by, an already known array of technical interventions. Hollon and Beck (2004), for example, discuss expanding cognitive-behavioral therapy (CBT) to include elements of psychodynamic and experiential therapy. The Casebook of Psychotherapy Incorporation (2006) by Stricker and Gold offers various examples of convergence of cognitive-behavioral interventions and multiple methods of psychotherapy. Beitman, Soth, and Good (2006) describe a three-tier psycho-social therapy with assimilative (first-tier) psychodynamic therapy that combines cognitive (second-tier) and behavioral (third-tier) interventions. Ryle and McCutcheon (2006) describe cognitive analytical therapy that incorporates psychoanalytic, cognitive, constructivist, behavioral, and Vygotskian sources. McCullough (2000) describes a cognitive-behavioral psychotherapy treatment framework that incorporates Bandura's (1977) theory of social thinking, Piaget's conceptualization of cognitive-emotive development (1954/1981), interpersonal procedures à la Kiesler (1996) and situational analysis, which is a problem-solving approach to real-life circumstances.

The Range of Effectiveness Associated with Cognitive Therapy

Comparative outcome psychotherapy studies for different psychological problems have generally led to the conclusion that treatments are broadly equivalent in efficacy. Unlike those who maintain that research reveals equivalent outcomes among therapies, however, CT disciples have asserted that their treatment is more effective than others across a variety of conditions and disorders.

Studies have shown that CT is effective in treating depression of various types, such as unipolar, major, minor, and acute depression. Positive findings have also been obtained in samples of endogenous depression patients, a subtype which is often thought to be psychotherapy refractory. CT appears to be effective in reducing depression and anxiety symptoms, and in increasing assertiveness in group and individual formats. A study by Ogles, Sawyer, and Lambert (1995) for the National Institute of Mental Health found that a significant number of clients who completed cognitive depression treatment showed reliable change to all outcome measures. Brown and Barlow (1995) have observed that CT greatly decreased somatic depressive symptoms, and depressed and nervous mood among alcohol users. In addition to these studies, Scogin et al . (1987) found that cognitive bibliotherapy reduced depression more effectively than either a control group with delayed treatment or a condition with attention—placebo – bibliotherapy. While this latter observation has not been reliably confirmed, even research that fail to reproduce these results indicate that patients that score fairly high on measurements of cognitive disability appear to have lower scores on assessments of severity of depression post-treatment compared to those with higher cognitive impairment. These findings strongly imply cognitive functions as important aspects of the improvement-related change processes, regardless of the treatment model used to address them.

CT also does well in pharmacotherapy comparisons. Most published trials found that CT is at least equal to, and sometimes superior to, pharmacotherapy

(Blackburn, Jones, & Lewin, 1986, 1996). In particular, studies have revealed that CT is equally or more effective than standard antidepressant drugs (Beck & Emery, 1985) and tends to have lower relapse rates (Hollon, 1996). Rush (1982), Rush, Beck, Kovacs, and Hollon (1977), Rush, Beck, Kovacs, Weissenburger, & Hollon (1982), and Murphy, Simons, Wetzel, and Lustman (1984) also discovered that CT was associated with more improvement than pharmacotherapy, and less attrition. In fact , patients were experiencing a higher dropout rate when researchers compared pharmacotherapy alone to CT. These studies also revealed that in improving depressive symptoms of hopelessness and low self-concept, CT exceeded pharmacotherapy. Even when CT is combined with pharmacotherapy, at discharge, patients tend to report significantly fewer depressive symptoms and negative cognitions than they do with pharmacotherapy alone (Bowers, 1990). CT appears to have a significant impact on the cognitive and vegetative symptoms of moderate and severe depression, as well as on the symptoms of mild and transitory depressive states.

In addition, CT has been found to be more effective than behavioral and interpersonal therapies. Gaffan, Tsaousis, and Kemp — Wheeler (1995) replicated a Dobson (1989) study which compared CT with other types of care. Although their study focused primarily on the effects of allegiance, CT was also reported to be superior to other forms of treatment, including behavioral therapy.

Clients who endorsed depression for both characterological and existential reasons responded better to CT than to behavioral interventions. Overall, there is strong support for the value of CT in treating depressed patients, but researchers are still uncertain as to the mechanisms by which this effect occurs.

CT also seems effective in the treatment of other types of disorders. CT is therefore effective in the treatment of anxiety disorders, particularly specific anxieties and phobias, and a host of other anxiety disorders and symptoms. Barlow, O'Brien, and Last

(1984) and Lent, Russell, and Zamostry (1981) found CT preferable to behavioral treatment in treating depressed patients. CT also promotes total abstinence among patients with alcoholism, both at the end of the treatment and during follow-up periods. Studies further suggest that CBT is effective in treating patients with eating disorders. In patients with bulimia nervosa, Fairburn, Jones, Paveler, Hope, and O'Connor (1993) used CT and observed significant and well-maintained therapeutic outcomes mirrored in all facets of functioning. In addition, Arntz and van den Hout (1996) found that CT achieved better effects in patients with panic disorder and a secondary diagnosis of either social or mood disorder compared with mediated relaxation by reducing the incidence of panic attacks. Furthermore, CT is useful in treating patients with problems marked by a lack of self-affirmation, rage, hostility, and addiction disorders.

In addition to research investigating the impact of CT on a range of patient issues and behaviors, a rising number of literature reports have attested to the potential of CT approaches to contribute to continuous symptom reduction. For example, a 1-year follow-up analysis by Kovacs et al. (1981) showed that self-rated depression for those who had undergone CT was dramatically lower than for those diagnosed with pharmacotherapy. Similarly, a 2-year follow-up analysis of patients diagnosed with CT, pharmacotherapy or a combination reported reduced relapse levels associated with CT. In addition, patients in the pharmacotherapy group had the highest rate of relapse following 2 years. Thus, although it is uncertain what characteristics of CT yield change in various classes of patients, it is evident that CT is successful, even more efficient than other types of care.

By virtue of the variety of conditions for which it is effective, CT has certain advantages over many other models, and in that sense has the making of a flexible and eclectic intervention model. However, this does not mean the CT practice is equally effective for all individuals. Research (e.g., Beutler, Mohr, Grawe, Engle, & MacDonald, 1991) reveals that CT 's efficacy is differently influenced by a variety of patient- and problem-specific qualities. Qualities such as patient coping styles, reaction levels, and problem complexity and severity, among others, may affect the way CT is applied.

One characteristic of the patient that has proven to predict the response of patients to CT is "coping style," the method that an individual adopts when confronted with anxiety-provoking situations, and that is typically seen as a trait-like pattern. CT was found to be most effective among patients exhibiting an extroverted, under-controlled, outsourcing style of coping. For example, Kadden, Cooney, and Getter (1989) evaluated alcohol patients and implemented cognitive-based social skills training as a procedure for preventing relapse through remediation of behavioral deficits in coping with interpersonal and intrapersonal drinking antecedents. Although CT was essentially as effective as other overall therapies, it was more effective than other interventions in patients that were fairly high on sociopathy or impulsivity tests. Beutler, Engle, et al . (1991) found this type of ATI, too. Depressed patients who ranked high on the Minnesota Multiphasic Personality Index (MMPI) outsourcing and impulsiveness tests reacted better to CT than to insight-oriented counseling. This pattern holds depressed patients as well as outpatients alike. Barber and Muenz (1996) have considered CT to be more effective than recovery approaches for people who escape their issues by outsourcing the blame. In addition, Beutler, Mohr, et al . (1991) and Beutler, Engle, et al . (1991) found that CT had significantly stronger effects on patients with outsourcing coping styles compared to customer-centered therapy or self-directed, supportive therapy. On the other hand, with customer-centered and self-directed therapy, internalizing patients did better than with CT. Similarly, the patient resistance traits and tendencies in the aforementioned studies differentiated the level of benefit achieved from the therapist-guided CT procedures and various patient-led or non-directive procedures.

Making Cognitive Therapy Systematically Fit Human Complexity

The main impetus for integration with psychotherapy comes from the evidence that no single psychotherapy school has demonstrated consistent superiority over the others. Instead, psychotherapy work on particular problems such as substance addiction or depression has largely contributed to the assumption that both methods have comparable average results (e.g., Lambert, Shapiro, & Bergin, 1986; Beutler, Crago, & Arizmendi, 1986; Smith, Glass, & Miller, 1980). Unfortunately, the non-significance of the main effects of treatment often draws more attention than the growing research body that shows significant differences in the types of patients for whom different aspects of treatment are effective.

Research, for example, shows that for patients with anxiety and depression symptoms:

(1) Experiential interventions are more successful than cognitive and behavioral therapy where there is inadequate initial anxiety regarding one's situation to encourage movement;

(2) Non-directive and paradoxical interventions in patients with high levels of pre-therapy resistance are more effective than guideline treatments;

(3) Interventions that address cognitive and behavioral improvements by risk management (e.g., Higgins, Budney, & Bickel, 1994) are more successful than insight-oriented therapy in impulsive or externalizing patients, but this result is reversed in patients with fewer externalizing coping types.

CT should be customized to suit the complex needs and preferences of people with a wide variety of conditions and diagnoses. In a recent study at our University of California Psychotherapy Research Lab, Santa Barbara, a number of guiding principles and strategies have informed the systematic application of tactics and techniques drawn from numerous theoretical perspectives. CT techniques can be used with virtually any patient; however, the greatest benefit is achieved with differential use of strategies or techniques, depending on patient dimensions such as coping style, type of problem, subjective distress, functional and social impairment, and resistance level.

For illustrative purposes, the rest of this section addresses some of the techniques and strategies that guide the application of CT techniques to internalize or outsource the patient, the resistant patient, and to manage the level of excitement. A detailed review of the aspects of patient – care matching (resistance/reaction level, coping methods, the extent of subjective pain, and functional impairment) and guiding principles, tactics, and collection of techniques can be found elsewhere.

Patient resistance typically bodes poorly for effective treatment unless it is skillfully managed. It is generally assumed that some patients are more likely to withstand therapeutic procedures than others. "Resistance" can be characterized as a dispositional trait and a temporary in — therapy state of oppositional behaviors (e.g., angry, irritable, and suspicious). It includes both intra-psychic (picture of self, health, and psychological integrity) and interpersonal factors (loss of interpersonal control or power enforced by another). "Reactance," an extreme example of resistance, is manifested by behaviors of opposition and uncooperative.

Three hypothesized factors determine the level of resistance or reactance potential of a patient. The first element concerns the patient's intrinsic appreciation in the individual right that is considered to be in peril. For example, one patient can appreciate the freedom associated with an unfixed schedule of time commitments, while another can be relatively comfortable with a schedule or routine imposed. The second element refers to the presumed proportion of rights that are challenged or lost. The addition of a therapy item that excludes or restricts a number of freedoms (e.g., a homework task that forbids drug use and involves social contact at an event for a certain amount of time) is likely to cause a high degree of reaction among resistance-prone, alcohol-abusing, and socially disconnected individuals. The third element concerns the degree of authority and control ascribed to the person or threatening force. The resistance generated by this factor comes from the preconceived notions of a patient and the differential allocation of authority to different professional occupations (clinicians, law enforcement officers, etc.). In comparison, direct encounters with a mental health provider can be beneficial in reducing or exaggerating such conceptions.

Resistance is readily recognizable, and differentiated recovery programs are conveniently designed for people with high and low resistance. However, the successful implementation of those plans is often quite another matter. It is difficult to surmount patient resistance to the efforts of the clinician. It requires the therapist to set aside his or her own resistance in recognizing that the oppositional behavior of the patient may infact, be iatrogenic. In a study in the Vanderbilt Study of Psychodynamic Psycho-therapy of experienced and highly trained therapists, none were able to work effectively with patient resistance.

Instead, therapists often responded to patient resistance by becoming angry, critical, and rejecting, which are reactions that tend to diminish patient willingness to explore problems.

In general, therapists should avoid open discord with patients who are highly resistant. CT 's collaborative relationship is an important antidote to resistance, and from the initiation of therapy this component should be emphasised.

Another common feature of CT, socratic interrogation or directed exploration, must be treated carefully to mitigate tendencies of resistance. A clinician should introduce this technique as a collaborative effort and generate feedback about the willingness of the patient to take part. The patient can also be elicited satisfaction with guidance and recommendations for exploration. Information about the level of resistance capacity of a patient can be learned from the history and actions of the patient during previous traumatic encounters or during the recovery process itself.

Research suggests that procedures that are non-directive, paradoxical, and self-directed produce better outcomes among patients with high resistance behaviors. Behavioral contracts created by patients and "suggested" homework assignments are non-directive strategies to help control resistant patients. For patients with extreme and persistent resistance, a "paradoxical intervention" might be considered in which the symptom is prescribed, or in which the patient is encouraged for a period of time to avoid change.

To put it simply, paradoxical interventions by discouraging it induce change (Seltzer, 1986). A paradoxical, non-directive intervention could involve the suggestion that the patient continue or exaggerate the symptom/behavior. A classic example of such an intervention could be the prescription of wakefulness for the insomnia complaining patient. An acceptable rationale for this type of intervention should be provided (e.g., "Your circadian rhythm is not set correctly. Staying awake will help reset your sleep cycle"). Non- or low-resistant habits suggest that patients are usually open to the therapist's external input or advice.

CHAPTER THREE

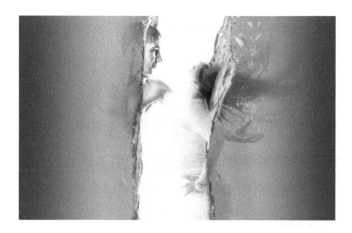

Overcoming Panic Attacks with CBT

The day-to-day tension and life's stresses can get very stressful. A lot of minor details tend to add up and ultimately lead to worry, anxiety, panic and even depression. It is only natural that the thoughts start to develop into a negative pattern from this point on. Changing the way of thinking, though, will help avoid such uncomfortable feelings. Here's some more information about cognitive behavioral therapy, which is considered by many to be the best panic attack treatment.

What Is Behavioral Cognitive Therapy?

The principle of cognitive behavioral therapy, or CBT, is that what people think will affect how they feel and behave emotionally. When under emotional distress, the manner in which someone sees and judges itself may become more negative. Therefore, CBT's aim is to help you begin to see the link between negative styles of thinking and mood. That will help you to regulate these thoughts more.

How It's Done

Cognitive behavioral therapy can be attributed to the best treatment for panic attacks, because it encourages you to develop positive thinking patterns. This happens in 3 steps:

Identifying Negative Thoughts-Situations with panic disorders are perceived to be more dangerous than they actually are. Shaking another person's hand, for example, may seem like life-threatening someone with a germ phobia. Though you may think this fear is irrational, it can be very difficult to identify your own irrational, fearful thoughts. One way to do that is to remind yourself what you felt before you began feeling nervous.

Challenging Negative Thoughts-The next step is to evaluate your thought-provoking fear. Here, you'll find out how realistic your concerns are. Ask yourself whether these thoughts are true, or an exaggeration. Weigh the pros and cons of thinking and the thing you 're scared of, and assess the likelihood that it will really happen.

Replacing Negative Thoughts-You should replace them with new thoughts, which are more rational and constructive, after you have recognized the bad ideas. Instead of saying you can't do anything to yourself, tell yourself you can. Whatever happens, tell yourself you 're going to be fine. Repeat reassuring and sedative statements until you feel calm. The more confident you hear, the happier you'll be.

There are two panic attack treatments-medication, and psychological therapy. Some people advocate the former while others advocate the former; some insist on a mix of the two. It's all getting a bit confusing so how do you know which course of treatment to follow?

Firstly, when it comes to panic attacks and anxiety problems, there is no particular solution that suits all. A cornerstone of effective therapy is that after a detailed study of the symptoms and when they occur, it is tailored individually to the person. This should apply irrespective of which panic attack treatment you choose to follow-and ultimately, it is your choice and you need to feel comfortable with that.

One of the most common approaches to psychology is that of cognitive behaviour therapy or CBT. Studies have shown that CBT is much more effective than medicine in the long run. To be more precise, six months after care ended, more patients who were diagnosed with CBT were panic-free than those on the drug. Another study showed that while medication might be effective in treating panic attack symptoms, the benefits stopped when the medication stopped. That is, people were forced to continue taking the drugs which then led to unpleasant side effects.

CBT therapy requires the therapist and, more importantly, the person seeking treatment to do the work and the commitment. It's not as easy as taking drugs a couple of times a day and the effects aren't seen so quickly, but if you compare a drug-free life free from panic attacks to taking medication for the rest of your life, then the benefits are obvious.

CBT 's focus is to get you to solve the problem yourself, so that you feel in control of your life again. This is very important as one of those suffering from panic attacks' biggest fears is that they have lost control of themselves, often to the extent that they feel they are losing their minds. The 'cognitive' part of therapy means to change the way you think through a very gradual process of desensitization.

Let's say, for example, that your first attack happened in a crowded room, perhaps at a party. Because the feelings were so intense and you were so scared you would never want to experience them again. So, you 're going out of your way to avoid that situation-you 're making excuses so you don't face a recurrence. But that means you stay by yourself at home while everyone else is having fun at the dance. Not an ideal situation.

So, desensitization involves first making very small steps to get you used to the thought of going to a party (cognition) and then getting you there (behaviour). Your first step may be as if you were going to get dressed. This is it. Just dealing with the feeling you are going to be one day is enough. This can last for several days until you feel comfortable thinking you 're going to a party. You take the next move, when you're ready, which might get dressed and then open the front door as if you're on your way out. That's it for step two. The third step when you are ready is getting dressed, opening and closing the front door. And so forth.

As you go through these steps at your own pace, you will also be taught how to deal with the conflicting feelings that you have. Instrumental here is controlling your breathing. Rapid breathing is often the catalyst for the other symptoms you experience during a panic attack so if you have techniques to keep your breathing rate stable then this could be the difference between a slight twinge of anxiety and a full-blown attack.

Many therapists agree that 10-12 sessions are enough for the majority of people to be able to manage their problems alone. Upgrades can be seen after the first five or six, and the person begins to feel confident they can regain control of their lives. A final step in the recovery process is to incorporate coping strategies in the event of potential stress trying to rear its ugly head. Armed with this knowledge, the possibility of panic attacks being a thing of the past is a very real one.

CONCLUSION

There are a number of options available for those looking for methods of overcoming the anxiety that can be considered "natural." What do those natural methods of relieving anxiety involve? These are basically anti-anxiety techniques and do not require the use of prescription medications or narcotics as a way to relieve the problem. These methods often prove far more healthy than what the overused anxiety treatment methods deliver. The cognitive behavioral therapy is one such method of overcoming anxiety.

Cognitive behavioral therapy isn't new. It has been used for decades by mental health professionals as a means of altering a person's behavioral choices that create mental health problems. In addition to being used as a way of reducing fear, cognitive behavioral therapy has also been used to treat many extremely severe mental health conditions. What does cognitive therapy involve, then? Here's a short outline of what's involved:

Cognitive behavioral therapy as a form of anxiety relief involves taking a two-pronged approach to the problem. The first half includes solving the neurological problems that cause fear. That is, they will examine the thoughts and psychological components of the problem. Basically, it will examine the mental triggers that cause anxiety, and then take steps to reverse the trigger effect.

The other side of the coin is the behavior therapy component for overcoming anxiety. This approach addresses the actual triggers associated with physical actions or activities which may cause an anxiety-based reaction. As with the cognitive therapy mental component, the aim of behavioral therapy is to modify one's trigger reaction to anxiety-causing activities.

Some will have legitimate questions regarding whether or not this form of treatment will lead to significant outcomes when it comes to managing anxiety. There's actually nothing to think about, as cognitive behavioural therapy has long been known to be a successful form of treatment. This is definitely not a new treatment methodology as it has been employed for many years to great success by psychologists and other mental health professionals. One of the main reasons why cognitive behavioral therapy works as a means to enhance one's ability to gain much needed anxiety relief centers on the fact that most people don't know what causes their anxiety. In a stunning number of instances, the person experiencing the problem is completely unknown to the triggers that cause the onset of anxiety , stress, or a panic attack. The ability to get to the core of what creates the anxiety is made possible through working with a therapist. From this, it becomes possible to overcome anxiety because it identifies the root of the problem.

It's an almost difficult challenge to conquer fear by going to the root of raising the tension of your life. Naturally, if you want to experience relief from anxiety, you will need to take control of all the things that cause you stress and anxiety in your life.

CPSIA information can be obtained
at www.ICGtesting.com
Printed in the USA
BVHW051506080321
601998BV00012BB/1453

9 781802 100655